HOW REHABILITATION RECONSTRUCTED MY MIND AND BODY

Virgil Reich

ISBN: 9781729747155

ISBN: 9781729747155

ABOUT THIS BOOK

This book is written to show why therapy should be done after any injury no matter how serious or simple. It will discuss the three ways of having therapy administered to you. It gives a complete procedure used by doctors my for my sixteen day in-hospital therapy after my broken hip surgery. It will give you an understanding of the different exercises and what part of your body is affected by the exercises. It lists different therapies and what ailment is affected. This book is in no way to be used to diagnosis or treat any medical problems. Consult your primary doctor before starting any medical regiment.

CONTENTS

ACKNOWLEDGMENTS

I want to thank everyone who gave me help in formatting and writing this book. Thanks to the therapists who taught me the exercises. They gathered my tools so I could film and use and then write about them. I also want to thank all the doctors, nurses and staff who were so friendly while providing me with outstanding service in the hospital part of my stay. A big thanks to Peggy, Lynette, Sabie, and Evan for proofreading and helping with the layout of the book.

CHAPTER ONE

THERAPY

When you have had an enormous medical condition or an accident you need therapy to regain your complete mind and body.   I realized this during two in-hospital therapies and four home health therapies. This is a story not about me, but about an incident in my life that has completely changed my mind thought about taking care of my body.

Occupational and physical therapy work hand in hand to improve our overall wellbeing.

Physical therapists are instrumental in helping to create a safe discharge plan. They help determine the appropriate discharge destination for the patient.

They go over the home environment with the patient and family to figure out what support and equipment the patient might need. "A lot of things the patient or the doctor doesn't think about are really important to us — mobility, feeding, positioning, prevention of falls and medication side effects."

Beyond the inpatient side of care, many hospitals are in the outpatient physical therapy business. As is the case with inpatient care, the type of patients physical therapists can serve in the outpatient arena go beyond the orthopedic and stroke recovery realms that usually pop to mind. They include patients who have diabetes, lymphedema, vestibular disorders and those who need continuing wound care.

The idea is that offering outpatient physical therapy as part of the hospital's care continuum helps to avoid readmissions and offers better patient care.

First a therapist knows what is best for your particular injury.   The thing that effects therapy most is willingness to keep doing it day after day.

There are three ways to have therapy administered to you.   The first and best is the in-hospital treatment.

That means you are admitted to a hospital therapy unit.

Each day you are scheduled to do certain exercises with a therapist assisting and guiding you through each exercise that effect your recovery.   They have at their disposal the necessary tools.

In-hospital therapy is necessary if your injuries have made certain movements and thoughts different or out of focus. The therapy will bring all those things back into original use as far as your body will allow.

In therapy there are those who teach you the vital needs of cleaning, dressing yourself, getting in and out of bed and chairs. They also have you do things to help with the movements of your arms, hand and fingers. These are the occupational therapist.

The other half of the therapy team is the physical therapist. They have you do exercises to build all your body muscles. For this reading both occupational and physical therapist will be referred to as physical therapy.

By the way; to assure privacy there will not be any individual or establishment names presented. Anything published is public knowledge or I have been given written permission to use.

CHAPTER TWO

MY SIXTEEN DAY IN-HOSPITAL THERAPY

To remove any misconceptions you have about physical therapy. I would like to take you through my sixteen day stay at the therapy unit.

The purpose of me needing rehab was a broken hip.

Oklahoma is our home of record. We moved to New Orleans with the idea of spending one half our time in Oklahoma and one half in New Orleans. Due to my medical conditions we are compelled to spend more time in New Orleans. We go for several weeks during the year to Oklahoma.

It was during one of our trips to Oklahoma on October 14, 2018 we were in Bossier City, Louisiana with a stopover for the night. About twelve am I decided to go to bed. I went into the bath room and I fell. The next thing I remember is an ambulance crew picking me up.

I was taken to a local hospital. They discovered I had a broken hip. In just a few hours the doctors replaced my hip. To be released from the hospital to return to New Orleans I had to find an in- hospital therapy unit that would accept me. My family called and found such a place. The next morning I was put in our van and transported to a hospital in New Orleans. This is really where my story about love, passion and dedication begins for the people of the therapy team who worked at reconstructing my mind and body to help speed up my recovery.

This is my daily workouts as best I can remember them. I also show the tools used and what the exercise is supposed to affect, again as best I remember.

Each day you are given three hours of therapy. The rest of the day is just like any other stay in a hospital with the nurses taking care of all of your personal needs. The first thing taught me was the easy and hard way to get out of bed. The second is how to get up from and how to sit down in a chair.

Here are my daily workouts.

Day 1: October 16, 2018

I arrived at the rehab center about 3 pm. After I was settled into my room the doctors started checking to determine just what was needed to start rehab the next day. I was given an x-ray and a sonogram.

The doctors, nurses and assistants were so friendly and efficient.

I then went to bed for the night with great anticipation of what was going to happen the next day.

Day 2: October 17, 2018

I was awakened about 7 AM in the morning. The occupational therapist was ready to give me a sponge bath and started talking about things that I could expect during rehab.

At 8 AM my breakfast was delivered. I ate then waited for someone to come get me and show me the procedures. When it was time, an attendant came and took me by wheelchair to the therapy room.

This was the first time I had tried to walk. I could not move my right foot or leg. I walked less than 10 feet dragging my right foot.

They had me lay on a mat. These are some of the exercises while lying on a mat:

Physical Therapy: Ankle Pumps

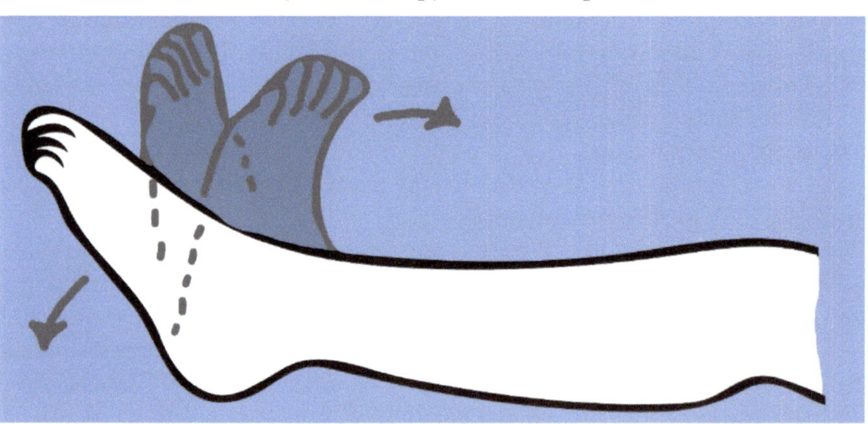

Point your toes down as far as possible. Then put the toes up stretching the calf as much as you can. You can also move your ankle in circles to help promote circulation. Do each leg 20 times.

<u>Physical Therapy: Quad Sets</u>

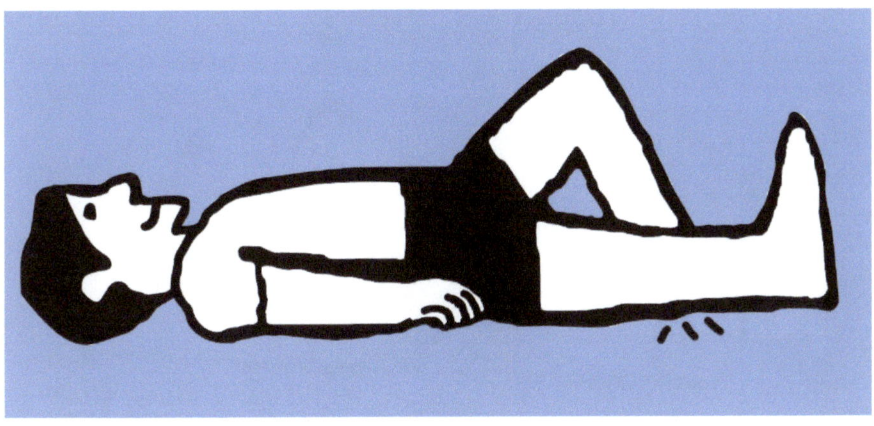

The quadriceps [quad] are the muscles on top of your knee. To tighten them, press your knee down to the mat. Hold for five seconds, then relax. Do 20 on each leg.

<u>Physical Therapy: Gluteal Sets</u>

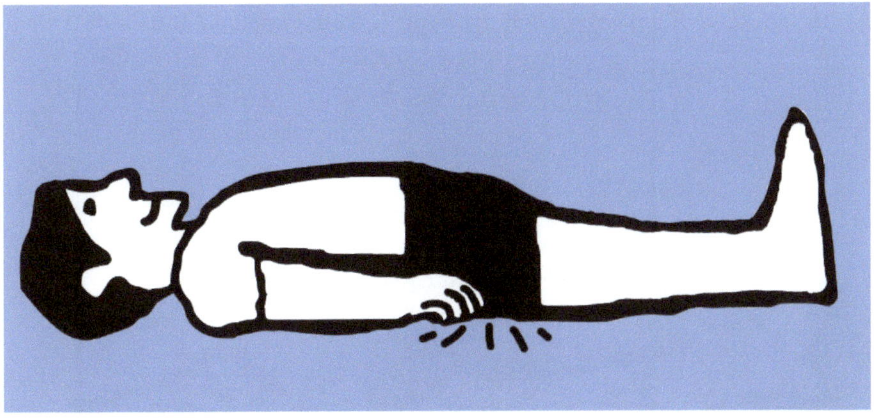

The gluteal muscle is located in your buttocks. By pinching your buttocks together as much as you can, you can help tighten your hip muscle. Hold for a count of five and then relax completely. Do 20 times.

Physical Therapy: Heel Slides

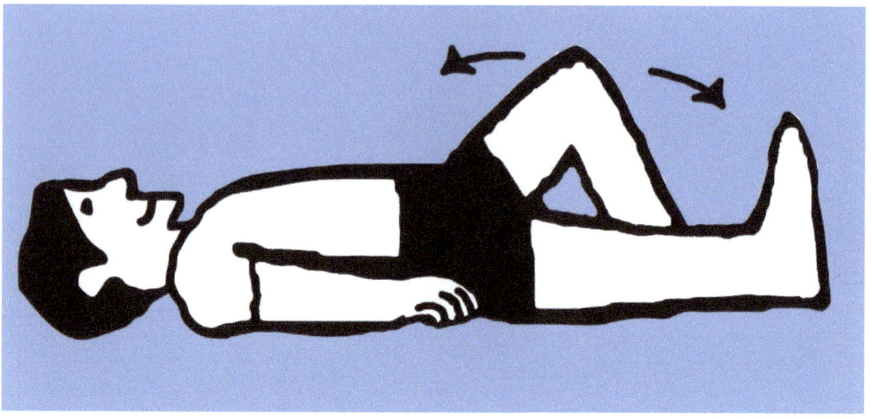

Bend your knees by sliding your heel toward your buttocks. Hold for five seconds, then slowly lower. Do 20 times.

Physical Therapy: Bend Knee Extension

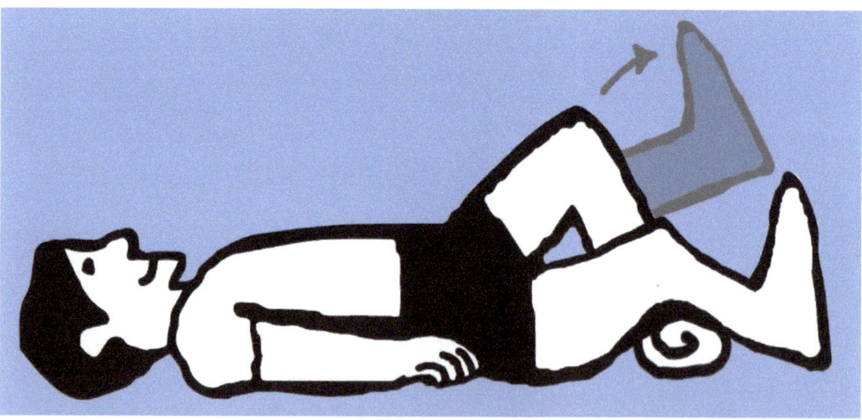

Place a towel under your knee. Lift your heel and then straighten the knee. Hold outstretched for five seconds, then slowly lower. Do 20 for each leg.

Physical Therapy: Hip Exercises

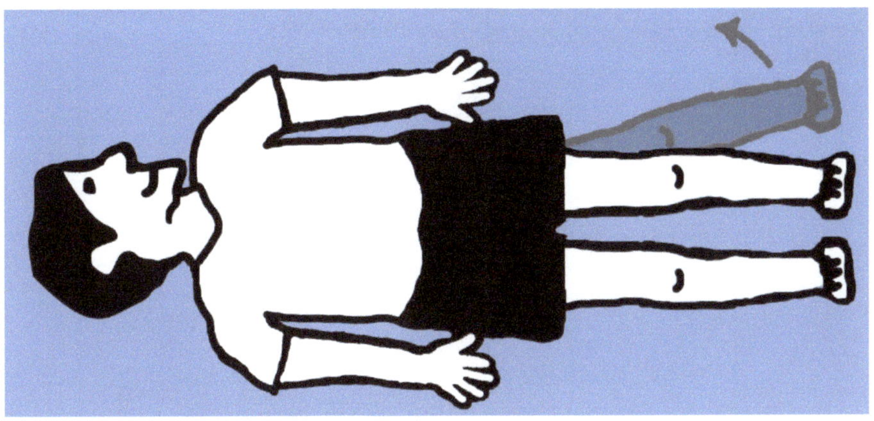

Lying on your back, spread your legs as far apart as possible, keeping your toes pointed to the ceiling. Slowly pull your legs back together without letting them touch. Do 20 times.

Physical Therapy: Parallel Bars

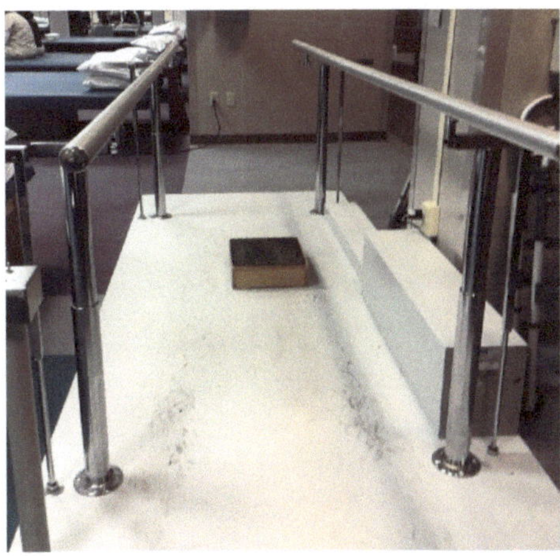

I then went to the parallel bars where I stood and moved my legs again from inside to outside. I also kicked forward and backwards. I then turned to stand straight with eyes closed to work on my balance.

Occupational Therapy: Bilateral Sander

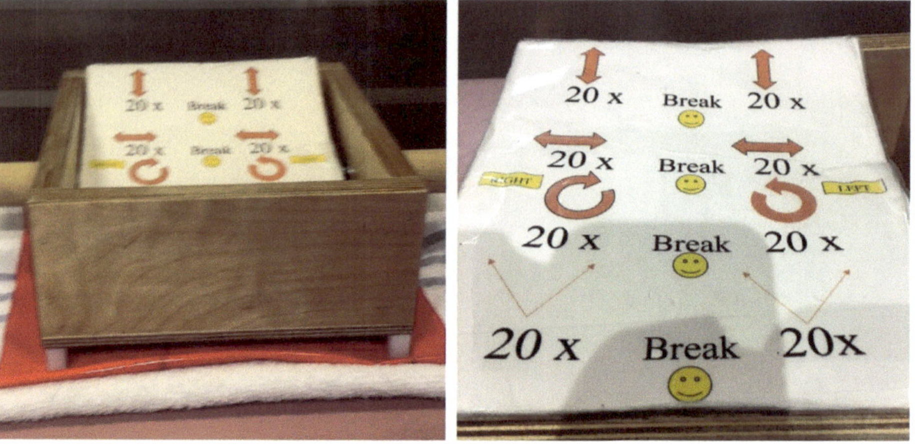

Now it was time for the occupational therapy. I started by doing a box sliding on the table, called bilateral sander. The Bilateral Sander is great for occupational therapy. It's especially helpful for work simulation tasks.

In the box is a note to show you which direction to move the box. There are 10 movements and each movement is repeated 20 times. I did it with a 1 pound weight in box.

Physical Therapy: Pegs in a Mat

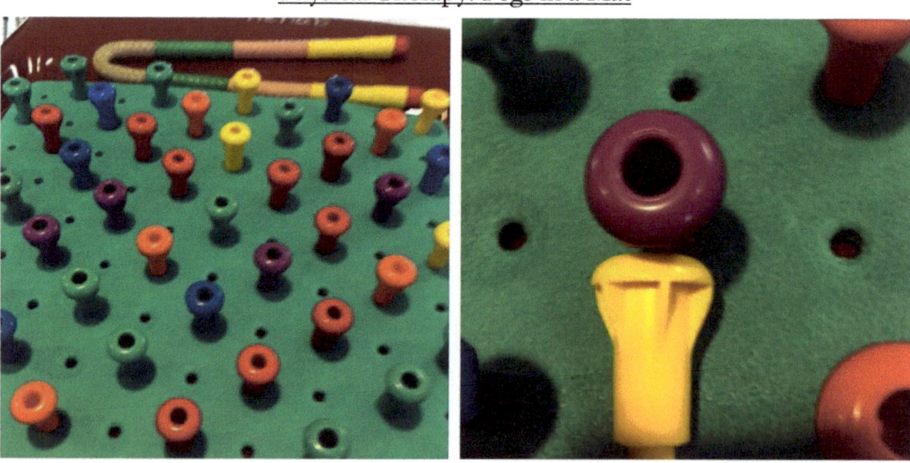

I then did pegs in a mat. The pegs are round and plastic like a drawer pull. The bottom is round and made to fit in a rubber mat with matching holes. There are 100 pegs. You have to put them all in the pad and then take them out. This exercise is to help strengthen and coordinate your fingers.

I was then taken back to my room for rest until the next morning.

Day 3: October 18, 2018

They got me up at 7 am to give me a shower and get me ready to start the day.

I walked 50 feet today. My leg was getting stronger. I did squats and pullups from a bar on the wall.

<u>Wall Bar</u>

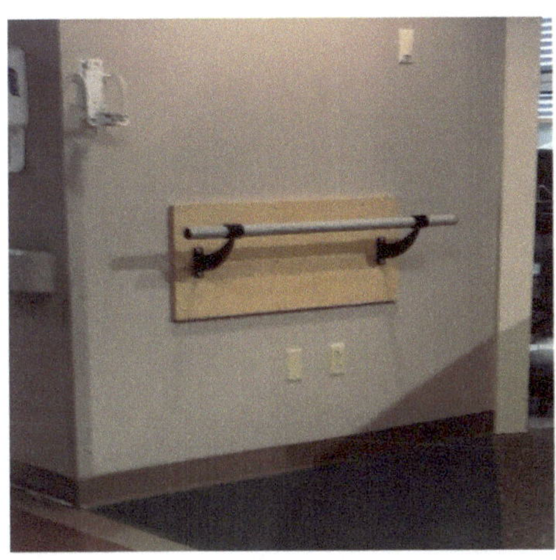

Each exercise required 20 reps each. This is to strengthen your arms and legs.

I worked on my balance on the parallel bars. Did 30 sidekicks with no weights. Did the bilateral sander with 2 pound weights.

Did rickshaw with 2 pound weight –10 x10.

<u>Can Do Rickshaw Rehab Exerciser</u>

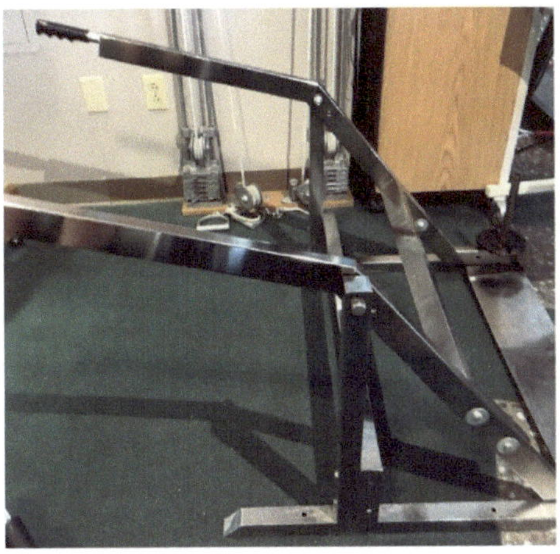

The Can Do Rickshaw Rehab Exerciser is designed for people who use a wheelchair to strengthen their arms and shoulder muscles. Stronger arms are needed for propulsion, transfer, and pressure reduction lifts. I walked 140 feet today.

On mat: did 20 toe stretches. Moved legs left to right 2x10. Pushed leg tight against mat. 3x10. Butt pull 2x20. Straightened legs 2x20. Bent legs at knee and pulled up as far as possible 2x20

Day 4: October 20, 2018

Arose early and did my wash down bath by myself. Ate breakfast and then was taken to therapy. I walked two time down the hallway and back.

On mat: did 20 toe stretches. Moved legs left to right 2x10. Pushed leg tight against mat. 3x10. Butt pull 2x20. Straightened legs 2x20. Bent legs at knee and pulled up as far as possible 2x20.

The pegs in the board was part of my exercises. I did the hand exercise twenty times each hand.

Hand Exerciser

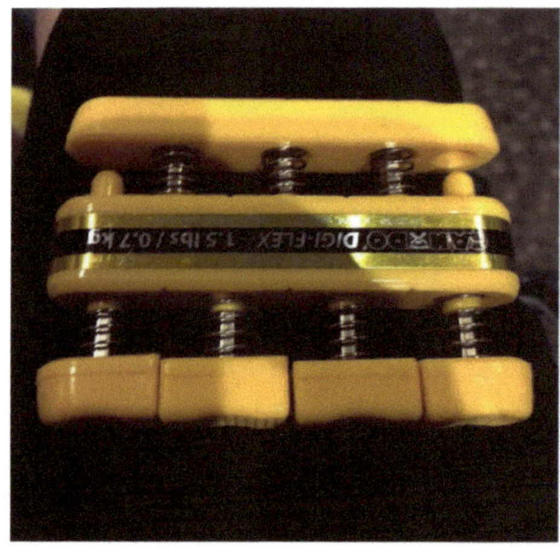

The hand and finger exercise is an excellent way to strengthen the hand. It also has a key for each finger to help them.

Day 5: October 20, 2018

Today I walked 280 feet. Drove wheelchair 140 feet. Did leg squats in wheelchair 2x15. Did pegs in mat. Got in and out of car. Walked up and down ramp. 1 time. Builds leg muscles. Placed clothes pins on bar.

<u>Car Loading and Unloading</u>

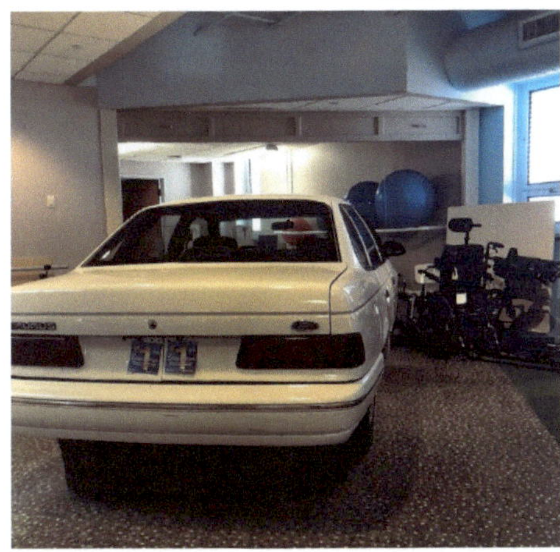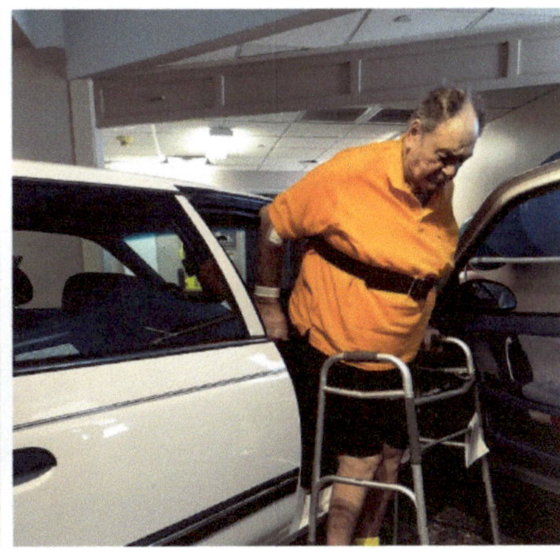

Day 6: October 21, 2018

No Therapy this day.

Day 7: October 22, 2018

This morning started great with my therapist coming to my room and helped me getting ready for the daily activities. Then breakfast was served and I was taken to the therapy room. Everyone in this facility are so nice and pleasant and caring.

During exercise I walked 640 feet. Drove wheelchair 160 feet. Got in and out of car. Did 30 leg stretches. Did legs from side by side -- 30 ea. Straightened legs then bend at knee -- 30 ea.

Day 8: October 23, 2018

My day started at 7am by a therapist coming to give me a sponge bath. In therapy today we did several different exercises. I walked 280 feet using my walker. To learn to use the wheel chair, I went by myself for 140 feet. I again did the plastic pegs in the mat. I used a small box called bilateral sander. Standing I played 2 games of connect four. The object of this is to help make your standing more stable.

Day 9: October 24, 2018

I was awaken at 7am so I could take my first shower since arriving at the facility. I did some occupational therapy. Like putting on my clothes, shoes and socks. This seems like a trivial thing. But you cannot put shoes and socks without bending unless you know what to do. And have the tools to do it. The therapy teaches you to do these things without bending forward. These are the tools we used.

Hip Kit

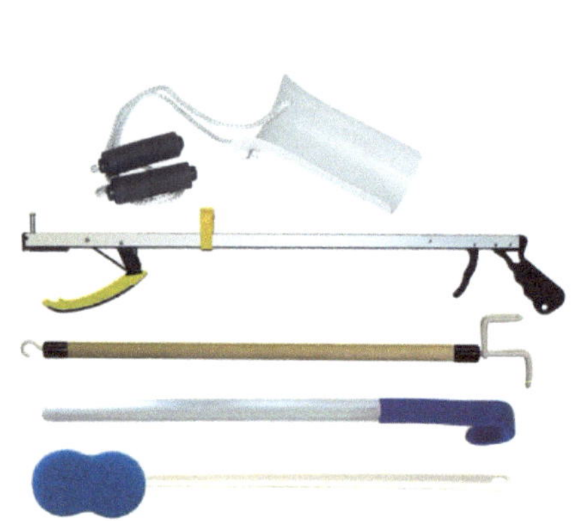 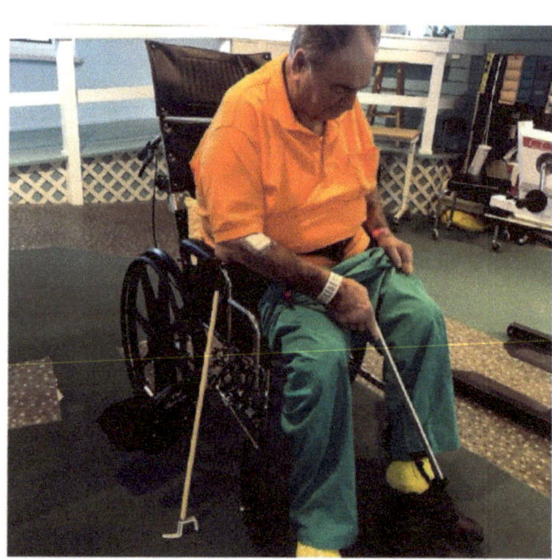

Two rotating grabbers and reachers. Both 32" and 19" Reacher grabbers are designed to rotate a full 90 degree for use both vertically and horizontally. 19" short grabber is ideal for where extra-long reach is not needed, for use in a car, wheelchair, or doing grocery shopping.

32" long reacher easily reach an item on top of shelves, or pick up dropped items. The nonslip rubberized jaw allows to pick up as small as a dime. 42" leg strap:

The Loop Leg Lifter, rigid and durable, is designed for repositioning the leg in a car, wheelchair or on a bed after hip replacement surgery, knee or back surgery, or leg injury. The lifter strap is strong enough to handle leg casts with ease.

28" Dressing Stick with a large vinyl coated "S" Hook to assist with putting on shirts, pulling up pants, skirts, or helping put on shoes or removing socks. Vinyl coated "C" Hook on opposite end for pulling zippers and shoelace loops. The Sock Aid allows to easily put on socks or stocking without bending over.

A 22" long Bath Sponge making bathing without bending and twisting easier.

A 24" long shoe horn is included to easily put on any type of shoe while standing.

Today I walked 520 Feet. I then practiced standing on a foam rubber pad to help my equilibrium. This took about 10 minutes. I then stood at a bar on the wall. I moved my legs from inside to outside 30 times for each. I then used my walker and went up a ramp that was inclined for about 30 feet, then I had to walk back down.

It was now lunch time. I had to be back to therapy at 2 pm. This time I lay on a training pad for the next exercises. I practiced getting in and out of bed. With a small round foam rubber cylinder placed under my feet I had to try touch the mat with my legs doing 30 per leg. Then a board was placed under my heels so I could move my legs from inside to outside. 30 per leg. This completed my therapy for the day

Day 10: October 25, 2018

Today was similar to most days. I Walked 820 feet. Then played bouncing ball with another patient. This is to help with balance.

On the parallel bars I did side to side kicks. I stood to help with balance.

<u>Dowell Exercise Bar</u>

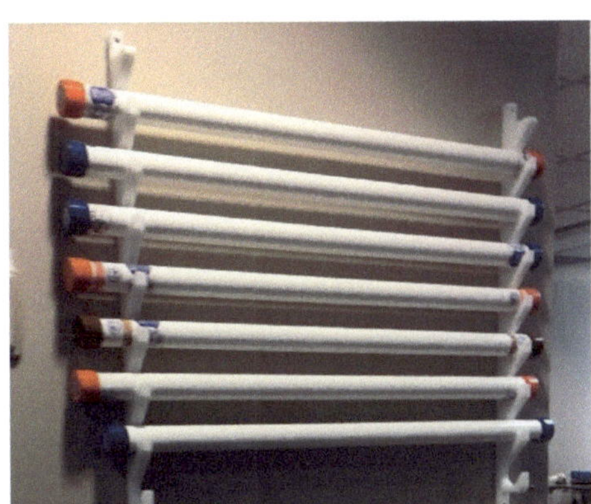

Color coded cap is different for each size for easy identification. Exercising with weighted bar helps to burn more calories, strengthen arms and legs, increase balance, flexibility and build core stabilization. Did bilateral sander 20 times each. Walked on ramp. Wheelchair pushups. 3x10 Rickshaw w/7pd weight- 10x10

Arm Bike

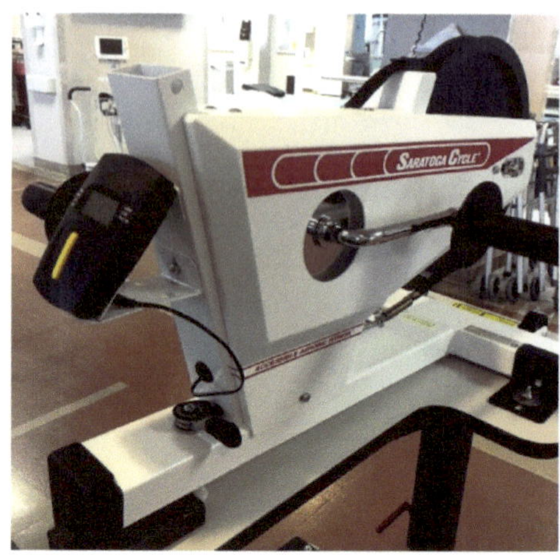 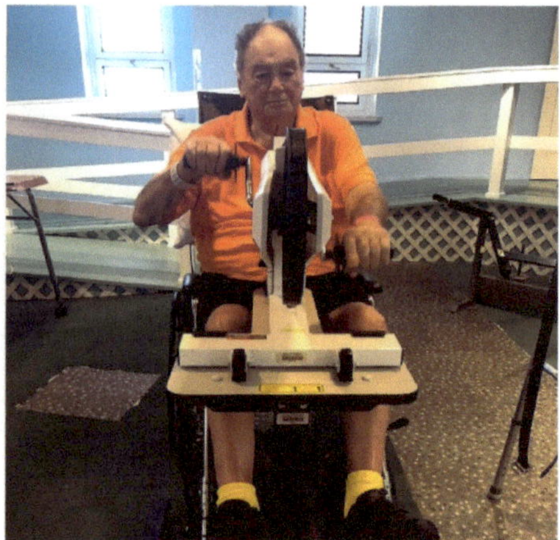

Magnetic mini stationary bike with handle for easy portability. Builds arm muscles. Do 3 times of 5 minutes each.

Day 11: October 26, 2018

Versatile Balance Pad

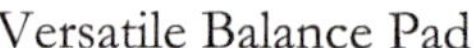

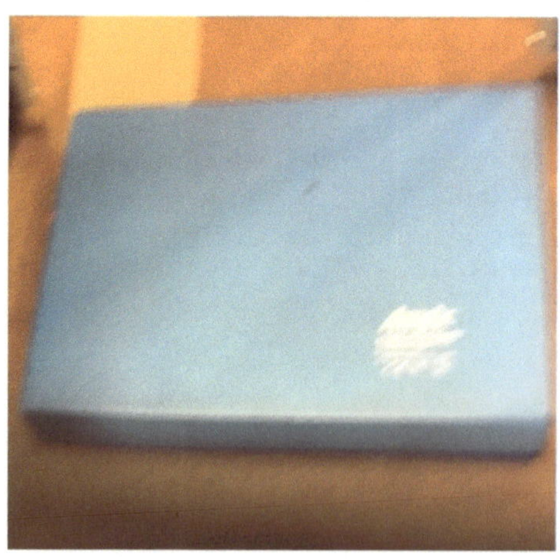

Designed with innovation, the balance pads are perfect for supporting in sitting or standing rehab activities and physical therapy exercises, balance training, yoga, and dancing. Strengthens body core and increase the difficulty levels of training like: squats, push-ups, lunges, spine balance, planks, sit-ups, yoga poses, step up & down and underwater balance. Convenient tool builds up bone resilience, muscles in a safe and stable way for whole body. It is a significant life jacket for the elderly in physiotherapy and people in injury recovery. Walked 750 feet.

Wobble Pad

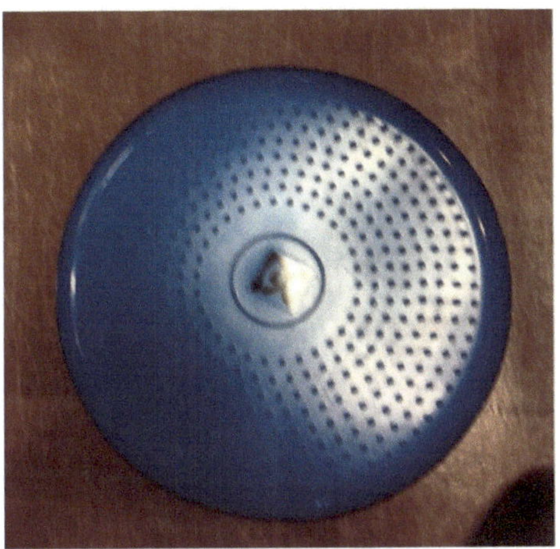

14in/35cm in diameter, large spiky dimples on one side (for standing), very small dimples on the reverse side (for sitting). Helps improve balance, coordination and flexibility; Good for active sitting, muscle strengthening, and joint stabilization.

I worked on putting on shoes and socks. Used Bilateral sander with 2 lb weight Rickshaw with 5 pound weight.   10x10. Arm wheel 5 min two times. In chair toe stretch 3X15. In chair leg kick out 3x15. Butt squeeze 3x15. Did the exercises on the mat.

Day 12: October 27, 2018

Without supervision, completed all the mat exercises twice.

Day 13: October 28, 2018

Without supervision, completed all the mat exercises twice.

Day 14: October 29, 2018

Breakfast arrived early. I was still eating when the therapist arrived to help me with a shower. We then worked on putting on my socks and shoes. We then went to the therapy room where I did the arm wheel 4 sets of 10. Next to the rickshaw with 10 pounds weight. Doing 10 sets of 10 ea. I practiced getting on and off the commode. I walked from one end of hall to the other and back 2 times. I walked on the ramp one time. I got in the car once. I did mat exercises. I worked on stability by hitting a balloon between 4 of us. I stood at my walker and worked on my balance.

Day 15: October 30, 2018

My day started by me doing a sponge bath and eating breakfast. Next I went down to the rehab room. I walked the length of the hall and back. I got in the car. I walked up and down three steps. The mat exercises were next except this time they put one pound weights on my ankles. I practiced getting on the commode and getting in the shower. The rickshaw had ten pounds weight. The bilateral sander had 3 pounds added. I also did the plastic knobs in the rubber mat. These added weights were pretty hard to do but was a gratifying feeling after I had finished.

Day 16: October 31, 2018

I got up early and had my sponge bath. Breakfast came shortly. After breakfast I took a nap. I was sleeping when Peggy and Lynette came to my room. Sabie was a little late, but we all went to the therapy room.

Today Peggy, Lynette and Sabie were here early so the therapist could tell and show them what was going to be needed when I got out of hospital therapy.

First I did sitting on the commode along with getting in the bath tub for a shower. Next I did the hand wheel. Then I got in the car. I also walked up the ramp and up three stair steps. I started walking and we did a bypass so they could see how I got in and out of the bed. I finished my walk. The family did a knee bend exercise together.

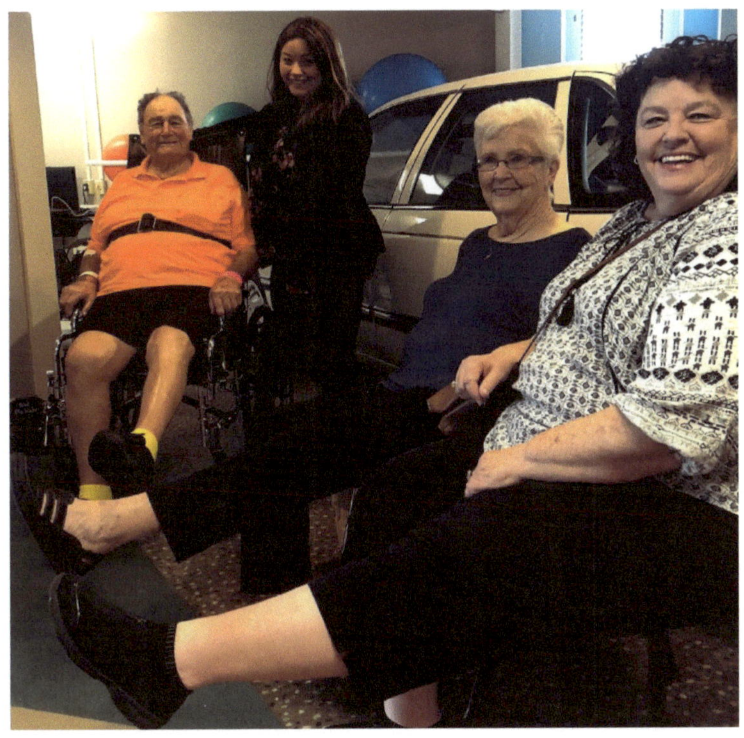

It is really rewarding having your family actually doing the exercises with you. We went to the training mat where I did all the mat exercises. I have now broken for lunch.

I finished the day off by doing the sander 20 times each exercise. Next I did the rickshaw 100 times with 15 pound weight added. I did the dowel bar 240 reps total.

I have relayed the therapy used to restore my body after hip surgery. Many, many of the same exercises and tools are used for every rehab patient. They are just adapted to each patient's needs. Many exercises used for other injuries are not listed because each patient is different. I just know after sixteen days of rehab the therapists have done an amazing job.   In the hospital part of my living was out standing with the most caring nurses, doctors and staff. My final evaluation shows that I am ready to be released from in-hospital rehab.

I was released from the therapy workout and the hospital on November 3, 2018. My next step is to have home health work with me.

CHAPTER THREE

THERAPIST TESTIMONIALS

When I was in rehab and decided to write this book I asked several of the therapist to please write why they got into the therapy field and what was most gratifying in what they did.

I was amazed at the answers I got. I have their permission to list them below. This is their statements word for word. I think you will see why caring therapist in every field of work are so dedicated.

I knew I wanted to work in the medical field. My mom is a nurse and I thought I wanted to do that too. My grandfather became ill with cancer. As I watched nurses care for him I realized that nursing was not for me. He had to come live with us for a little while. A physical therapist started coming to the house to see him. At this time I realized that this was what I wanted to do. I began volunteering with the physical therapist and eventually become a physical therapist myself. Inpatient rehabilitation has always been my favorite place to work. I love helping people who have found themselves in unexpected situations. Life sometimes throws things at us and we need a little help from the people around us, friends, family and healthcare workers to get back on track. It is a joy to give people care and physical therapy treatment so they may return home and get back to their regular life. H. C.

Rehab is a unique setting in this profession because of how well you get to know your patients. You get to see their progress day in and day out as well as spend one and a half hours per day with them. The gains they make both physically and mentally/ emotionally are more drastic in this setting than any other. The appreciation these patients tend to have is greater than you can imagine. B. C.

I love giving patients and families "Hope"! Sometimes rehab is about learning a new way of doing things and adjusting to the new norm. I love supporting patients through that journey. My greatest joy is seeing a patient work through their fear and anxiety and watching them get their smile back! That usually means that things are going well. R. G.

I started off wanting to make films when I was in college, but then I started working as a direct service worker and began being exposed to pediatric pt. Slowly but surely I became enamored how pt's assist/enabled these kids in their mobility. I like helping them regain their independence. V. C.

I decided to go into rehabilitation specialty since I have a genuine compassion and love for people. There is nothing more rewarding than to work with patients recovering from an accident or medical issue and to see that individual regain their independence again. It is truly an honor to work with patients and have positive outcomes. W. M.

Working in inpatient rehab for over sixteen years now has been very rewarding and inspiring. One of my favorite things is learning about what obstacles and trials patients have overcome in their lives. I also love to see the recovery that the patients make during their stay in rehab. I can't go without mentioning all the patients who are still in love after fifty + years of marriage and how they still take care of each other so much after all these years just warms my heart. C. C.

When deciding to become a therapist in the medical field I was more concerned with my future earnings. After working with people for a while I found how rewarding it was to help people regain the strength and self-esteem. Everyone who has an accident needs some therapy. M. B.

CHAPTER FOUR

HOME HEALTH

You have seen how my in-hospital therapy was such a success. You have read the remarkable stories of my therapist in their own words. It is now time for the second phase of therapy: Home Health.

Home health is used to continue your therapy after you are discharged from in hospital care.

A qualified and certified nurse will be assigned to check you every week to determine if any new medical problem exist or seem to be developing.

An occupational therapist will visit you to determine if you need their assistance with anything in your normal day to day chores.

A physical therapist will evaluate you to determine which exercises is best for your condition. The therapist will have you do the exercises in their presence. These exercises are to be done on a timely basis as prescribed by the therapist. Your improvement will continue faster only if you follow the instructions.

I am now home and doing very well. I now have home health visiting me.

The nurse has checked my medical condition.

The occupational therapist visited to make sure I was capable of taking care of my personal needs by myself.

My physical therapist came by to evaluate what therapy exercises I needed. I am following their advice and I am daily doing the exercises they recommended. My therapist is presently visiting me two times each week.

CHAPTER FIVE

OTHER THERAPIES

Self-Therapy

After home health releases me I will enter the third part, called self-therapy. After the first two therapies you are left to your own desires of what you want to do. The best is to continue with a daily exercise as recommended by your therapist. This is the most difficult for one reason: YOU PROBABLY WILL NOT CONTINUE. If you take the attitude *I will do this*, then you will succeed.

Cognitive Behavioral Therapy

Cognitive Behavioral Therapy often called CBT is a type of therapy that helps people look at and change their thoughts and behaviors. For instance if you believe you need to stay drunk to cope with life. The therapist will help you learn that it is not necessary to be drunk to succeed.

Dialectical Behavioral Therapy

Dialectical Behavioral Therapy or DBT is a type of therapy that helps people work on acceptance and change. DBT got its name because of the dialectical nature of these two things. They seem to be opposites. How can you accept something and change it at the same time? This therapy helps people with an addiction, suicidal. The therapist helps you do this by helping you tolerate and sit with uncomfortable feelings or situations that cannot be changed. Simultaneously the therapist will help you have the confidence to change the thoughts, feelings, or situations that can be changed.

Motivational Interviewing

Motivation Interviewing is a type of therapy that was specifically developed for people with addiction. In motivational interviewing the therapist and the patient are working together with one another. The therapist encourages and motivates the client in order to help them change. In this type of therapy it is thought that there are motivational blocks that get in the way of recovery. By having a therapist who is aligned with the client and there to motivate them it helps them break through those motivational blocks.

Eye Movement Desensitization and Reprocessing

EMDR is a type of therapy that was developed for people who are coping with post-traumatic stress and anxiety.

Patients are asked to think of the event or stimuli that induces anxiety. Then they follow the clinician's finger with their eyes.

According to Scientific American, this is thought to work because it allows the two hemispheres of the brain to connect and process information in a new way. During rapid eye movement (REM) sleep the eyes do a similar action. It is thought that this is one of the ways that our brain helps us process information. Mirroring these eye movements that you have in REM sleep is thought to have a similar effect.

Family Systems Therapy

Family systems therapy asks the client to take a look at how their problems fit within the larger family system. This is done by having families come in and work on interpersonal communication among other things. Family members are asked to try and understand one another and relate to one another in new ways. This perspective views the family as an emotional unit. Each person in the family is looked at in relation to the whole.

Equine Therapy

Equine therapy is a type of therapy where clients interact with horses in conjunction with a therapist. Increasingly popular with holistic rehab centers, it is thought that interacting with an animal in this way can improve communication, anxiety, trust, and self-esteem. It is important to note that equine therapy is done in conjunction with other types of therapy and it not usually used by itself.

Speech Therapy

Speech therapy addresses speech, language, cognitive-communication, and oral/feeding/swallowing skills to identify types of communication problems (articulation; fluency; voice; receptive and expressive language disorders, etc.) and the best way to treat them.

The therapist will help with improving coordination of speech muscles through strengthening and coordination exercises, sound repetition and imitation. Improving communication between the brain and the body through visual and auditory aids such as mirrors and tape recorders.

Hopefully after reading this list you have a better idea of the types of therapy that are out there and how they might be used. The best way to figure out what works for you is to be informed about what they are and what they are usually used for. The list above features types of therapy that many inpatient treatment centers are now offering as they have been found to be helpful for people struggling with addiction or co-occurring disorders.

To show you how powerful physical therapy is to providing a new way of life, I would like to relay you a true story as told to me by my physical therapist some time ago.

The therapist was sent to a young lady's house. This is what she found. A young lady in her thirties who had been in bed two years. She said she could not even sit up. Her mother had to do everything for her. She had to feed, bathe, change her diaper and did anything else she needed. As the therapist talked to her, she was convinced she could help her. She told the lady. "We are going to get you up and walk today." The lady stated there is no way I can or will walk. The therapist said if you don't let me help you right now, I am leaving and not coming back. The lady agreed and they started with her. By the time the therapist left, not only was the lady sitting, but together they walked across her room and back to the bed. Her mother could not believe her eyes. This shows how powerful therapy can be to mend both the mind and body.

YOU
MAY FORGET
WHAT YOUR
THERAPIST
SAID,
BUT YOU
WILL NEVER
FORGET
HOW THEY MADE
YOU FEEL !!